Balance Exercises for Seniors

A Guide to Easy and Effective Exercises to Improve Balance and Prevent Falls

Lana Cochran

Introduction

Welcome to "BALANCE EXERCISES FOR SENIORS." This book is your guide to a healthier and more confident senior life.

Balance is like a secret ingredient in our lives. It keeps us steady, helping us stay upright physically and emotionally. This book is all about discovering the magic of balance and how it can make our lives better.

For seniors, it is a secret weapon that helps you live life to the fullest.

In these pages, we will show you why balance matters, how it can prevent falls and injuries, and why it is the key to your independence. We will guide you through step-by-step exercises that are easy to follow, helping you improve your balance and stability.

But this book is not just about exercises. It is about feeling better, moving more freely, and enjoying life with confidence. By the end, you will not only understand the importance of balance, but you will also have the tools to make it a part of your daily life.

So, let us begin this journey to rediscover your balance, boost your well-being, and embrace a more independent and active senior life.

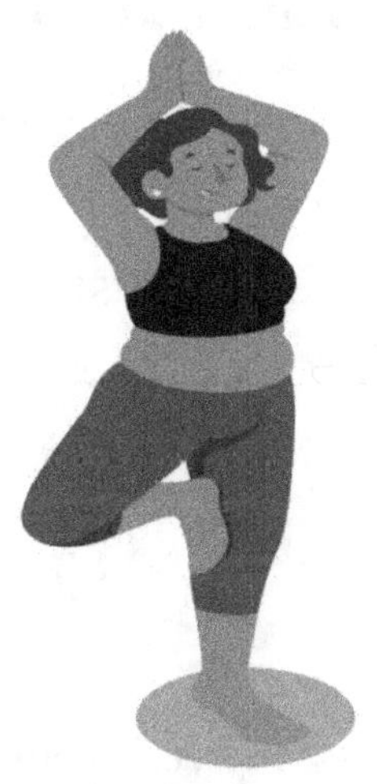

Importance of Balance for Seniors

Balancing our bodies helps us stay steady on our feet. For seniors, balance is like a superhero power that keeps them from falling. It is especially important because, as we get older, our balance can become less dependable.

Reducing the Risk of Falls and Injuries

Falls can be a real danger for seniors. They can lead to injuries that take a long time to heal. When seniors practice balance exercises, they become less likely to fall, like having a safety net that catches them if they wobble.

Promoting Overall Well-being and Independence

Imagine being able to move around freely and without fear. That is what good balance can do. It is not just about preventing falls; it is about feeling confident and independent. When seniors have good balance, they can continue doing the things they love for longer.

Benefits of Balance Exercises

Improved Stability

Think of stability like having a solid base. Balance exercises help seniors become more like a sturdy tree with deep roots. This means you are less likely to wobble or lose your balance in everyday activities.

Enhanced Coordination

Coordination is like a dance between your body parts. When you practice balance exercises, it is like your body is learning to dance better. You will find it easier to move gracefully and control your movements.

Increased Confidence

Imagine feeling sure of yourself as you move through life. Good balance can do that. When you know you are less likely to stumble or fall, your confidence grows. It is like having a secret superpower.

Better Posture

Posture is how you hold yourself. Balance exercises help seniors stand up straight and tall. Good posture does not just look better; it can also help you breathe easier and feel more comfortable.

Greater Mobility

Mobility is the ability to move freely. When you work on your balance, you are like an athlete training for a big race. You become more agile, making it easier to go where you want, when you want.

Practicing balance exercises, you will enjoy these amazing benefits and lead a more active, confident, and stable life.

Safety Precautions

Consultation with a Healthcare Professional

Before you begin your balance exercises, it is a bit like getting a green light from a wise coach. Talk to a healthcare professional to make sure these exercises are safe for you. They will give you personalized advice based on your needs and health.

Use of Proper Footwear

Imagine wearing the right shoes for the right activity. Just like a hiker wears sturdy boots, you will want footwear that supports your feet during balance exercises. It is like having the right gear for your adventure.

Clearing the Exercise Area of Potential Hazards

A safe space to practice is like a clean, tidy room. Make sure your exercise area is free of things that could trip you up. It is easier to balance when there is nothing in your way.

Having a Support System in Place

Even superheroes have sidekicks, and you should too! Having someone nearby, like a family member or a friend, while you are doing balance exercises can be comforting. They are like your safety net in case you ever feel unsteady.

Following these safety precautions, you will be on the path to balance success while staying safe and secure.

Types of Balance Exercises

STATIC BALANCE EXERCISES

Stand on One Leg

- Imagine you are a flamingo, gracefully standing on one leg.

- Find a sturdy surface to stand on, like a non-slip floor.

- Lift one foot slightly off the ground while keeping your knee slightly bent.

- Hold your arms out to your sides or place your hands on your hips.

- Focus on a spot in front of you to help maintain balance.

- Try to hold this position for 10-30 seconds.

- If you wobble, it is okay – just try again. Over time, you will get better.

Heel-to-Toe Walk

- Pretend you are walking on a tightrope, like a circus performer.

- Find a clear, open space.

- Begin by taking one step forward with your heel touching the toes of your other foot.

- Place your foot in front of the other, like a straight line.

- Take a step forward, heel-to-toe, without losing balance.

- Repeat this walk for about 10-20 steps.

Tree Pose

- Stand tall with your feet hip-width apart.

- Shift your weight onto one leg while bending the other knee.

- Reach down and place the sole of your bent foot against your standing leg, either below or above the knee, but avoid pressing on the knee itself.

- Bring your hands together in front of your chest, like you are in prayer.

- Focus on a point in front of you to help with balance.

- Hold this pose for 15-30 seconds, then switch to the other leg.

Static balance exercises like these are great for building a strong foundation in balance and stability. Keep practicing, and you will become more confident on your feet.

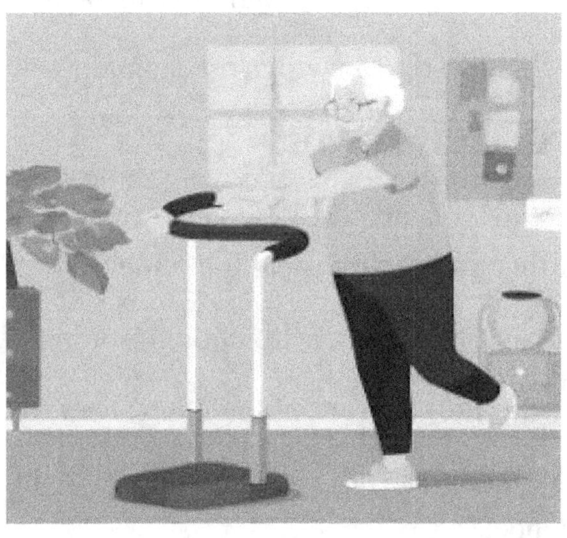

Dynamic Balance Exercises

Leg Swings

- Imagine you are a pendulum, swinging back and forth.
- For balance, find a sturdy support, such as a chair or a wall.
- Stand up straight with your feet together.
- Hold onto the support and swing one leg forward and backward, like a pendulum.
- Try to swing your leg higher with each swing.
- Do this for 10-15 swings on each leg.

Tandem Walk

- Pretend you are walking on a tightrope again, but this time, without taking wide steps.
- Find an open space with enough room to walk.
- Put one foot in front of the other, heel to toe.
- Take slow, steady steps without losing your balance.
- Walk forward for about 10-20 steps.

Side Leg Raises

- Imagine you are a graceful dancer lifting your leg to the side.

- Stand next to a sturdy surface, like a counter or a chair, for support.

- Stand up straight with your feet together.

- Lift one leg out to the side as far as you can comfortably can.

- Lower your leg back down.

- Repeat this for 10-15 leg lifts on each side.

Dynamic balance exercises challenge your coordination and agility. These exercises can help you feel more in control of your movements and reduce the risk of tripping or stumbling. Keep practicing enhancing your dynamic balance.

Balancing on an Unstable Surface (e.g., Foam Pad)

- Imagine you are conquering a balance challenge on a soft cloud.

- Place a foam pad or cushion on the ground.

- Stand near a stable surface or have someone nearby to hold onto if needed.

- Step onto the foam pad with one foot, then the other.

- Try to balance on the uneven surface. You will feel wobbly – that is okay.

- Hold this position for 15-30 seconds, then switch to the other foot.

Sensory Integration Exercises

- Sensory integration is like training your brain and body to communicate better.

- Find a comfortable spot to sit or stand.

- Close your eyes to rely on your other senses.

- Gently lift one leg and move it forward, backward, or to the side.

- Try to touch your toe to the ground without putting weight on it.

- Repeat this movement 10-15 times on each leg.

Proprioceptive training challenges your body and mind to work together, making you more aware of your movements and surroundings. These exercises improve your ability to balance in various real-life situations. Keep practicing to build your proprioception.

Sample Balance Exercise Routine

Gentle Neck Stretches

- Stand or sit up straight with your shoulders relaxed.

- Gently tilt your head to one side, bringing your ear toward your shoulder. Hold for 15 seconds.

- Slowly return your head to the center and repeat on the other side.

- Next, tilt your head forward, bringing your chin toward your chest. Hold for 15 seconds.

- Bring your head back to the center and tilt it backward, looking upward. Hold for 15 seconds.

- Finally, gently turn your head to one side, looking over your shoulder. Hold for 15 seconds and repeat on the other side.

- These neck stretches prepare your upper body for balance exercises.

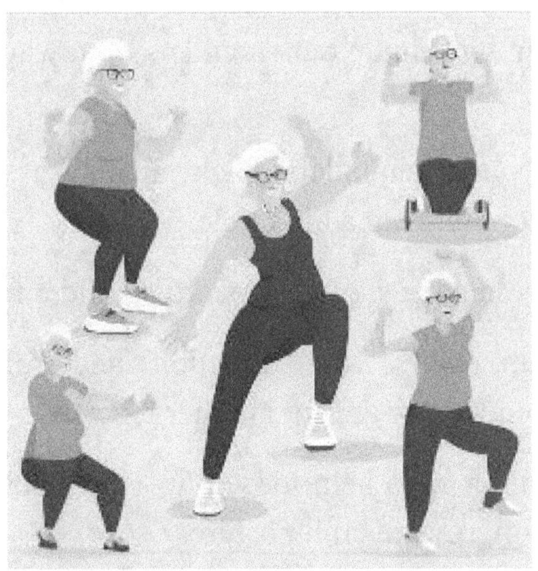

Shoulder Rolls

- Stand or sit up straight with your arms relaxed by your sides.

- Begin by lifting your shoulders up towards your ears.

- Roll your shoulders backward in a circular motion, making a big circle.

- Complete ten slow, backward shoulder rolls.

- Then, reverse the direction and roll your shoulders forward for another ten rolls.

- Shoulder rolls help loosen up your upper body and improve overall posture.

Ankle Circles

- Sit on a chair or stand with your feet flat on the ground.

- Lift one foot slightly off the ground while keeping the other foot firmly planted.

- Begin to rotate your raised ankle in a circular motion.

- Complete ten clockwise circles and then ten counterclockwise circles.

- Switch to the other ankle and repeat.

- Ankle circles help improve ankle mobility and prepare your lower body for balance exercises.

Including ankle circles in your warm-up routine can further enhance your ankle flexibility and stability, which is essential for balance exercises.

Static Balance Exercises (e.g., Standing on One Leg)

- Find a clear, safe space to practice.

- Stand up straight with your feet hip-width apart.

- Shift your weight onto one leg while gently bending the other knee.

- Hold your arms out to your sides or place your hands on your hips for balance.

- Concentrate your attention on a fixed point in front of you.

- Gradually lift the non-supporting foot off the ground.

- Try to stand on one leg for 10-30 seconds.

- If you wobble or lose balance, do not worry – it is a part of the process. Repeat on the other leg.

Dynamic Balance Exercises (e.g., Leg Swings)

- Find a stable surface or support to hold onto.

- Stand with your feet hip-width apart.

- Swing one leg forward and backward like a pendulum.

- Start with smaller swings and gradually work up to larger ones.

- Aim for 10-15 swings on each leg.

- Maintain a steady rhythm and controlled movements.

Proprioceptive Training (e.g., Foam Pad Exercises)

- Place a foam pad or cushion on the ground.

- Ensure you have nearby support, like a sturdy surface or someone to assist if needed.

- Step onto the foam pad with one foot, then the other.

- Balancing on the uneven surface, focus on maintaining stability.

- Aim to hold this position for 15-30 seconds on each foot.

- As you become more confident, you can increase the challenge by closing your eyes or moving your arms.

These main balance exercises encompass static and dynamic balance along with proprioceptive training. Regularly practicing these exercises will help you build a strong foundation in balance, coordination, and stability, leading to greater confidence and mobility in your daily life.

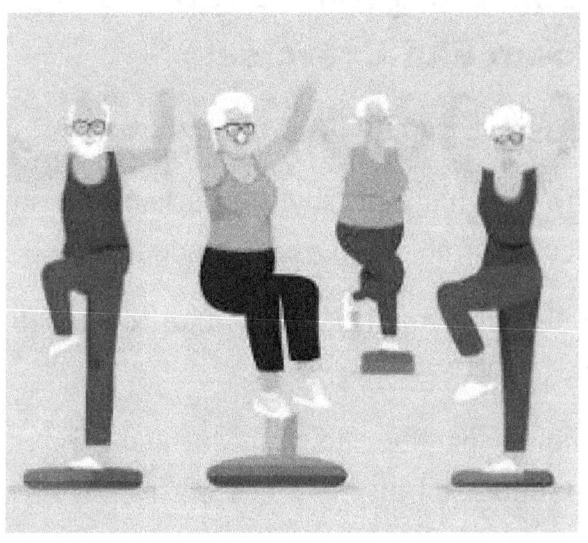

COOL-DOWN AND STRETCHES

Calf Stretches

- Find a wall or a stable surface for support.

- Stand facing the wall, with one foot about a foot's length away from it.

- Place your hands on the wall at shoulder height for balance.

- Step the other foot back, keeping it straight, with the heel firmly on the ground.

- Bend your front knee and lean your body toward the wall.

- You should feel a gentle stretch in your calf muscle.

- Hold the stretch for 15-30 seconds, then switch to the other leg.

- Repeat the stretch 2-3 times for each leg.

Hip Flexor Stretches

- Stand up straight with your feet hip-width apart.

- Take a step forward with your right foot, and a step back with your left foot.

- Bend your right knee to create a lunge position.

- Keep your upper body upright and engage your core.

- You should feel a stretch in the front of your left hip.

- Hold the stretch for 15-30 seconds, then switch to the other leg.

- Repeat the stretch 2-3 times for each leg.

Upper Back Stretches

- Stand or sit up straight with your shoulders relaxed.

- Clasp your hands together in front of you.

- Round your upper back by pushing your arms forward while tucking in your chin.

- You should feel a stretch between your shoulder blades.

- Hold the stretch for 15-30 seconds.

- Release the stretch and gently roll your shoulders back and forth a few times.

- Repeat the stretch 2-3 times.

This cool-down and stretching exercises are essential for helping your body recover and maintain flexibility. They reduce the risk of muscle soreness and help promote overall well-being.

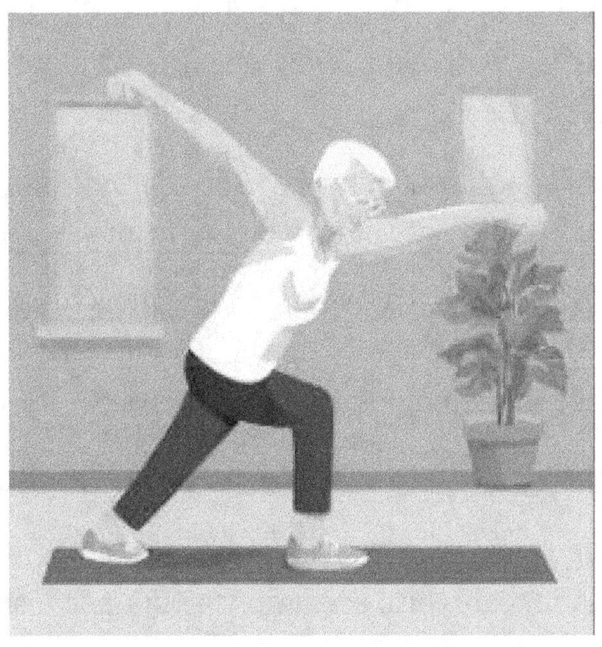

Progression and Adaptation

Gradual Increase in Difficulty

- Just like leveling up in a video game, gradually making exercises more challenging is the key to improvement.

- Start with the basics and, as you get comfortable, make the exercises a bit harder.

- For example, if you have mastered standing on one leg with your eyes open, try it with your eyes closed.

- You can also increase the duration of the exercise or add light weights to make it more demanding.

- Remember, progress does not have to be fast; it is all about moving at your own pace.

Incorporating Balance Challenges

- Life is not always steady, so it is a good idea to mimic real-world scenarios in your exercises.

- Try balancing on a less stable surface, like a wobble board or a cushion.

- Practice your balance while doing activities you enjoy, like gardening or dancing.

- You can even add elements of multitasking, like turning your head or reaching for an object while balancing.

- By introducing these challenges, you will become better equipped to handle balance in various situations.

Tracking Progress and Setting Goals

- Imagine your fitness journey as a road trip with milestones. It is essential to keep track of your progress and set achievable goals.

- Consider maintaining a balance exercise journal to record the time, duration, and how you felt during each exercise.

- Set specific, measurable goals, like being able to balance for a minute or improving your leg swing height.

- Celebrate your achievements, no matter how small they may seem. It is your journey, and every step forward is a win.

- Regularly revisit your goals and adapt them as you improve.

Progression and adaptation are like the gears that keep your fitness engine running. They ensure you keep challenging yourself while maintaining a sense of accomplishment and motivation on your balance improvement journey.

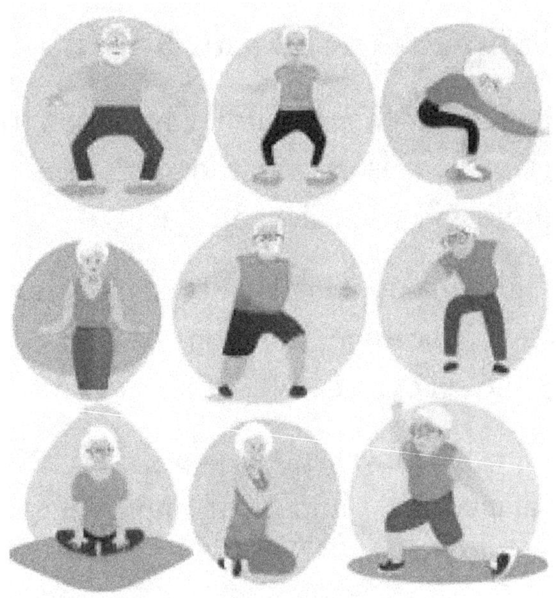

Motivation and Consistency

Group Classes and Social Engagement

- Balance exercises can be more enjoyable when you do them with others.

- Consider joining group fitness classes designed for seniors or balance-specific programs.

- Social engagement not only makes your workout fun but also provides a support system.

- Interacting with like-minded individuals can boost your motivation and make exercise a social event.

Keeping a Training Journal

- Just like a diary for your fitness journey, a training journal can be a valuable tool.

- Record your balance exercises, progress, and any challenges you face.

- Tracking your improvements, even small ones, can be incredibly motivating.

- It is a great way to stay organized and visualize your accomplishments.

Celebrating Achievements

- Celebrate your accomplishments, no matter how minor they may appear.

- Every day you maintain balance a little longer or perform an exercise a bit better is a victory.

- Treat yourself to small rewards or acknowledge your accomplishments with positive self-talk.

- Celebrating achievements keeps you motivated and excited to continue your balance journey.

Staying motivated and consistent with your balance exercises is crucial for long-term success. By engaging with others, keeping a training journal, and celebrating your achievements, you will create a positive environment that encourages you to keep working towards better balance and well-being.

Balance Exercises During Daily Activities

- Your daily routine is a fantastic opportunity to sneak in some balance exercises.

- While brushing your teeth, try standing on one leg for a minute.

- When waiting in line or chatting on the phone, practice heel-to-toe walking.

- Use everyday tasks as moments to fine-tune your balance without disrupting your schedule.

- These small, consistent efforts can make a big difference in the long run.

Household Modifications for Safety

- Make your living space a safe haven for balance.

- Remove clutter and obstacles that could cause you to trip.

- Install handrails or grab bars in areas like the bathroom or stairways.

- Secure rugs to prevent them from sliding.

- Creating a safe environment is like an insurance policy for your balance.

Regular Eye and Vision Check-ups

- Good balance starts with clear vision. Regular eye check-ups are crucial.

- Your vision helps you navigate the world around you with confidence.

- If you experience vision changes, consult an eye care professional for guidance.

- By ensuring your vision is in top shape, you will maintain your balance and safety.

Integrating balance into your daily life is not just about exercise; it is about creating a balance-conscious environment. By incorporating exercises, making safety modifications, and looking after your vision, you will enhance your well-being and independence in your everyday activities.

Local Fitness Classes and Senior Centers

- Your local community offers fitness classes tailored to seniors.

- Senior centers are excellent places to connect with others and find fitness programs.

- Inquire about classes focused on balance exercises and overall wellness.

- Trained instructors can guide you through exercises and ensure you are in a safe and supportive environment.

Online Tutorials and Videos

- The digital age brings a wealth of resources to your fingertips.

- Look for online tutorials and videos designed for seniors' balance exercises.

- You can follow these exercises from the comfort of your home at your own pace.

- Online resources are a convenient and accessible way to maintain your fitness.

Community Support Groups

- Joining a community support group can provide motivation and companionship.

- Many senior-focused organizations or social groups have balance exercise programs.

- Sharing your journey with others and gaining insights can be both educational and inspiring.

- Community support groups offer a sense of belonging and encouragement.

These resources for seniors can help you on your balance improvement journey. Whether you prefer in-person classes, online guidance, or the camaraderie of a support group, there are options available to fit your needs and preferences.

Conclusion

Reiterating the Importance of Balance for Seniors

- Never underestimate the significance of balance in your life as a senior.

- It is the pillar that keeps you steady, helping to prevent falls and injuries.

- Maintaining good balance contributes to a higher quality of life and overall well-being.

Encouragement to Start and Maintain a Regular Balance Exercise Routine

- It is never too late to take that first step toward better balance.

- Today is the perfect day to begin and commit to a regular balance exercise routine.

- The journey may have its challenges, but the rewards are well worth it.

Aging Gracefully and Independently through Balanced Well-being

- Picture yourself aging gracefully, confident, and full of vitality.

- By embracing balance exercises, you are investing in your future independence.

- With dedication and consistency, you can savor the joys of an active and balanced life.

In the end, the path to balanced well-being is within reach. Your journey to better balance is not just about maintaining your physical equilibrium; it is about claiming your independence and cherishing the freedom to enjoy life to the fullest.

THANKS FOR READING